Immunizing Children

a practical guide
Second edition

Richard Mayon-White
Consultant in Communicable Disease Control, Oxfordshire

and

Judith Moreton
District Immunization Coordinator & Health Visitor, Oxfordshire

RADCLIFFE MEDICAL PRESS

© 1998 Mayon-White and Moreton

Radcliffe Medical Press Ltd
18 Marcham Road, Abingdon, Oxon OX14 1AA, UK

First edition 1997

Every effort has been made to ensure the accuracy of these guidelines, and that the best information available has been used. This does not diminish the requirement to exercise clinical judgement, and neither the publishers nor the authors can accept any responsibility for their use in practice.

British Library Cataloguing in Publication Data

A catalogue record for this book is available from the British Library.

ISBN 1 85775 219 8

Typeset by Advance Typesetting Ltd, Oxfordshire
Printed and bound in Great Britain by Biddles Ltd, Guildford and King's Lynn

Immunizing Children

a practical guide

Second edition

Contents

Acknowledgements

This book would not have been written without the stimulus of people who:

- were anxious parents
- asked questions that we thought had obvious answers
- were reluctant to vaccinate and thereby protect children
- found defects in existing guidelines.

We repay this stimulation by not naming those who provoked us – to be honest, there are too many to remember them all.

This book is an update of *Immunizing children* by Sue Sefi and Aidan Macfarlane (Oxford Medical Publications, 1989) and we thank them and their publishers for permission to use their text.

We are grateful to Dr David Elliman, our colleagues in the Oxford Vaccine Group, the Oxfordshire Community Health NHS Trust and the Oxfordshire Health Authority for their advice and encouragement.

We thank Radcliffe Medical Press for their help in making such a success of the last edition.

Any errors in this book are our responsibility, and we shall be grateful to readers who point them out to us.

AUTHORS' NOTE

All four countries in the United Kingdom have similar patterns of childhood infectious diseases and therefore share immunization policies. The national vaccination policy is decided by an expert committee, the Joint Committee on Vaccination and Immunization (JCVI). The JCVI advises the Department of Health, the Welsh Office, the Scottish Office of Health and the Department of Health and Social Security (Northern Ireland). For simplicity, we use the term Departments of Health (DoH) for these government departments. For the most part, we have used the infectious disease statistics for England and Wales because they reflect our own experience, but there are no significant differences in Scotland or Northern Ireland.

DEDICATION

We dedicate this book to the memory of Sue Sefi who died in November 1996.

1

Introduction

The immunization of children is the single most cost-effective form of prevention and a positive health benefit to children. At a Royal College of Nursing conference on immunization against infectious disease in May 1986, it was stated that it is 'every child's right to be immunized'. The World Health Organization (WHO), in its document *Health for all*,[1] has clearly stated its aim of eradicating from Europe, by the year 2000, poliomyelitis, measles, neonatal tetanus, congenital rubella, and diphtheria. Initially targets were set at 90% uptake of immunization by 1990, but this was raised to 95% by 1995 as the only effective means of achieving the ultimate aim of the WHO, that of eradication of disease. The goal of eradicating these infections from Europe by, or soon after, 2000 is still achievable. With this aim, the WHO has initiatives in all its regions, with strategies to maintain high levels of immunization, national immunization days, enhanced surveillance of vaccine-preventable diseases and periodic checks that there is no accumulation of people susceptible to infection. It looks as though it will be possible to eradicate polio from the whole world by the year 2000.

Enthusiastic and knowledgeable health workers can achieve very high immunization levels in the communities in which they work.[2] Immunization uptake levels can be used as a measure of the effectiveness of the primary health care team, as each member delivers consistent advice, and contributes to the smooth running of a co-ordinated service.

DEVELOPMENT OF SAFE AND EFFECTIVE VACCINES

There has been much adverse publicity about the development of vaccines in recent years, with allegations that new vaccines are not properly tried and tested. It is important to address these concerns, not just of parents but often, misguidedly, of some health professionals. Vaccines are 'prescription-only medicines' which means that their use is regulated. The regulations cover the manufacturing standards, the recommendations on who should be vaccinated, and any special precautions that may apply. No vaccine is licensed in this country until it has been tested for efficacy, safety and acceptability. Trials done in other countries contribute to the information used in the licensing procedures, but the assessment carefully considers the applicability of the data to the groups of people for whom the vaccine will be prescribed. There is a careful assessment of predictable risks in comparison with foreseeable benefits to the population, and within that assessment is the overriding concern of the interests of the individual subject.

Before the process begins, there is the initial recognition of the need to protect both the individual and the community from mortality and morbidity of a particular infection. There then follows the laboratory development of the vaccine and the tests to ensure that the vaccine is safe to give in clinical trials.

Phase I

The vaccine is tested on small numbers of healthy adult volunteers, to determine both the safety and overall tolerability in human beings.

Phase II

The aim of the second phase of vaccine development is to demonstrate that the new vaccine is safe and effective in producing antibodies, and thus preventing the condition in the population for which it is employed. For example, the early Hib vaccines were not acceptable in the UK because they were ineffective in producing adequate antibody response in the population most at risk from Hib disease – the under 2s. It was only as the vaccines were further developed to protect that population that the DoH considered their overall use. Part of the second phase is also concerned with dose, age ranges for future use and the schedules required to produce an adequate immune response.

Phase III

During this phase more extensive trials are conducted on both the short- and long-term safety and efficacy of the vaccines. These trials are conducted within the population group for which they are intended, e.g. Hib vaccine in the under 4s, and pneumococcal vaccines amongst the susceptible elderly population.

Licensed vaccines

Even after a vaccine has been granted a licence and is in general use, surveillance continues to detect less common reactions or problems associated with the vaccine. For example, it was this continued surveillance which detected that the Urabe strain of mumps, used in certain MMR vaccines before September 1992, was responsible for causing vaccine-related meningo-encephalitis, and which led to those particular vaccines being taken off the market. This ongoing process is maintained by the reporting of any adverse reaction to the Committee on Safety of Medicines, using the yellow card system in the back of the *British National Formulary* (BNF).

The status of a licensed vaccine is important. It means that the vaccine has been properly tested, and has been shown to be relatively safe and effective. 'Relatively' refers to the risks of the disease in unvaccinated people. All licensed vaccines used in the UK have to be assessed by an independent national committee in Britain, and all have been through similar assessments in other countries. The production of licensed vaccines is carefully monitored and samples of new batches are independently tested.

A few vaccines available on a 'named patients basis' have not been licensed. This implies that they are not for general use. They are intended for special purposes, e.g. children at unusually high risk of a disease, or for those working abroad in a tropical climate. The message is 'use with caution'.

Population protection

The next step in the immunization of children is the administration of the vaccine to the entire population at risk. To achieve this, all health professionals involved in immunization must be both knowledgeable about the procedures and confident about the benefits. It is essential that the advice and information they deliver to parents should be consistent, accurate and reliable, thus allowing the parents to make a properly-informed decision.

This practical guide has been written to ensure the proper completion of this second step. It is in line with the 1996 *Immunisation against infectious disease*, produced by the DoH,[3] but is written in a practical and easily accessible form. It is for those 'in the field' who are directly responsible for giving immunizations – general practitioners, health visitors, school health nurses, practice nurses, clinical medical officers and district nurses. It is written so as to be understandable to parents.

Immunization policy

Immunization policy is based on scientific evidence of benefit and risk. It was as a result of this that routine smallpox innoculation ceased in the early 1970s when it became apparent that the risks from the disease were limited to importations, and that the risks from side-effects of the vaccine far outweighed that of the disease.

Immunization in the 1970s did not have a high priority; first because there were no clear guidelines for determining who had overall responsibility for co-ordinating and providing the service and second because the evidence-based information for those immunizing was minimal.

Because of these factors and the scare in 1974 linking pertussis vaccine and infant brain damage, continuing research and surveillance is now recognized as an important part of ensuring that immunization policy remains appropriate.

Research and surveillance

A well-defined, appropriate study design is critical to answer the question under investigation. In addition, ethical review and approval is also required and before publication all papers are subject to peer review. Most importantly, *no* research findings can stand alone and the weight of evidence is increased by other studies.

Occasionally a study which has set out with one research question may find other unexpected results which cannot be ignored. For example, clinical trials in 1996 into a combination vaccine of diphtheria, tetanus, acellular pertussis (APV) and Hib vaccines, unexpectedly and inexplicably found that APV somehow reduced the production of acceptable antibody levels (Unpublished data. Personal communication, Oxford Vaccine Group). Until this problem is resolved, this combination vaccine cannot be used routinely because it has failed to satisfy efficacy and acceptability criteria.

Surveillance

Following the introduction of a new vaccine, surveillance continues to ensure that there are no unforeseen problems, such as side-effects previously unrecognized, or a decline in efficacy.

Surveillance is now recognized as an important and on-going part of immunization policy and is supported by the sharing of international data and careful observation by independent scientific experts. These experts include the World Health Organization (WHO), the Joint Committee on Vaccination and Immunization (JCVI), and the committee of the Medicines Control Agency.

PRACTICAL USE

This book is intended to be practical with margins to be used for notes by the user. Spaces have been left for you to fill in the following information:

■ your local 'phone numbers showing whom to contact with queries on data collection (p. 45)

■ your local 'phone numbers showing whom to contact with queries concerning an immunization problem (p. 45).

Amongst much other essential information are chapters which provide the answers to the most common problems and to the questions most frequently asked by parents.

2
Why we immunize

The purpose of immunization is threefold. First it offers protection to the individual child and prevents them suffering from serious infections which can either pose a substantial risk of mortality or carry a high risk of morbidity and long-term sequelae. Second is the prevention of substantial outbreaks of infectious disease; by achieving high levels of immunization uptake; 'herd immunity' helps protect the approximate 1% with genuine contraindications to immunization. These include those children undergoing treatment for malignant disease such as leukaemia. Third is the worldwide eradication of a lethal disease. This has already been achieved with smallpox, and in 1994 the WHO declared the Americas free from poliomyelitis. Mass campaigns are being conducted in many countries of the world, including the UK, as part of a concerted programme to rid the world of measles and poliomyelitis.

Immunity can be induced either actively or passively, against a variety of bacteria and viruses.

ACTIVE IMMUNITY

Active immunization can be defined as an encounter with one or more antigens which provokes an antibody response so that the child develops immunity to a disease. This is achieved either by natural infection or by exposure to attenuated, live micro-organisms, inactivated micro-organisms, purified parts of micro-organisms or to their products. The effect of active immunity is usually lifelong.

PASSIVE IMMUNITY

Passive immunity is short term, and is acquired either from antibodies crossing the placental barrier from the mother, or from an injection of normal human immunoglobulin. The former offers protection of up to a year, for example, in the cases of mumps, measles and rubella; whilst the latter only offers protection for a few weeks. Normal human immunoglobulin may be used to protect individuals exposed to specific infections, such as hepatitis A, or to protect exposed individuals undergoing immunosuppressive treatment.

Specific immunoglobulins, such as tetanus, hepatitis B, varicella–zoster and rabies contain higher levels of antibody and are used to protect at-risk individuals; for example, unimmunized individuals with tetanus-prone wounds and pregnant women in contact with chickenpox who have no detectable antibodies.

The present immunization policy in the UK offers vaccination to all children to protect them against the following diseases:

- diphtheria
- pertussis (whooping cough)
- tetanus (lockjaw)
- poliomyelitis
- *Haemophilus influenzae* type b (Hib) meningitis and epiglottitis
- measles
- mumps
- rubella (German measles)
- tuberculosis (BCG vaccine).

In addition, there are circumstances in which selective vaccination is offered to children:

- hepatitis B vaccine: at birth to babies whose mothers are hepatitis B antigen positive, or in childhood if a member of the same household has hepatitis B

- BCG (bacille Calmette–Guérin): to neonates whose parents have come from places where tuberculosis (TB) is common, e.g. the Indian subcontinent and Africa; and in childhood if the child has an increased risk of close contact with an adult with TB (household contact or travel to or from places where TB is common)

- varicella vaccine: to children with severe immunosuppression from leukaemia or organ transplantation

- pneumococcal vaccine: to children over 2 years of age who have homozygous sickle cell disease or have had the spleen removed (trauma, spherocytosis), diabetes, chronic renal disease or chronic liver disease

- meningococcal A&C vaccine: to children who have close contact with a case of group C meningococcal disease, or children travelling to places where group A meningococcal disease is epidemic.

For the last 50 years, the vaccination policy in the UK has maintained consistently that immunization of children is a matter for parental choice. It has been suggested that there should be a legal requirement for children to be vaccinated before starting school, as in some other countries. A legal requirement in the last century for children to be vaccinated against smallpox caused public protests in England, and failed to ensure that the majority of the population was vaccinated. In the UK, good health education and well-managed vaccine services based in primary health care can achieve high vaccination rates. It is the responsibility of all health workers to ensure that parents are given correct and up-to-date information, to enable them to choose wisely.

Information about immunization develops at an increasing pace. Health workers must keep up-to-date, and be prepared to change some of their own views and advice to parents. It is important for health workers to recognize that contraindications may change. In the 1970s, for instance, one misconception was that asthma and eczema were contraindications to measles immunization. In the early 1980s, many doctors thought that children with a family history of epilepsy in first-degree relatives should not be immunized against whooping cough. However, this opinion has now changed as it is recognized that this medical condition does not increase the supposed risks from the vaccine. As medical knowledge expands, health workers need to be able to find further information.

There is also a need to recognize the small but increasing number of parents who either refuse vaccination in general, or who are selective about which immunizations they will accept. An expanding body of literature from this country and abroad suggests that the advice offered by health professionals is one-sided, only stressing the benefits and largely ignoring or underplaying the hazards.

There are a few community groups who have unusual views or special beliefs about vaccines. By congregating unvaccinated (and therefore unimmune) people, the children in these groups are at risk from imported infection. Outbreaks of polio and measles have occurred in some of these groups, in contrast to very little or no disease in the rest of the population.

Every child eligible for immunization should be offered that protection. All the diseases that we immunize against may have severe consequences for those who are unprotected.

DIPHTHERIA

In 1940, just before the introduction of the diphtheria vaccine, there were 46 281 cases of diphtheria in England and Wales, with 2480 notified deaths in a year. By 1957 the figures had dropped to 37 cases with six notified deaths in a year. In the 10 years from 1987 to 1997, the total number of cases was 55, with one death of a 14 year old with no record of immunization who had visited Pakistan.

Although there has been a dramatic fall in incidence and mortality, immunization levels for diphtheria must be kept above 95%. The causative organism may be present in some symptomless carriers, and cannot be eradicated.

Diphtheria is caused by a bacterium, *Corynebacterium diphtheriae,* which produces a toxin that inflames the membranes of the nose and throat, blocking the larynx and so obstructing the airways. Antibiotics are effective, but if antitoxin is not given quickly a toxin produced by the bacterium will attack the heart and nervous system. Complications include:

▪ heart damage

▪ paralysis (which may recover)

▪ death (in up to 10% of all cases, the 1–4 years age group being the most vulnerable).

Diphtheria increased in Eastern Europe, especially in Russia, after 1990 because of poor vaccination uptake. Because of this, low-dose booster doses of diphtheria vaccine are recommended for children in their mid-teens.

TETANUS (LOCKJAW)

Tetanus vaccine was introduced into the basic course of immunization of infants in 1961. From 1960–9, 200–300 cases (all age groups), with about 27 associated deaths a year, were reported in England and Wales. Notifications have since fallen to less than 15 a year. In the five years from 1992 to 1996, there were only 30 notifications, principally in older women who had not been vaccinated when young. Tetanus in children has become extremely rare in the UK. Internationally, the target is to eradicate neonatal tetanus by vaccinating mothers in pregnancy.

Tetanus spores are present in soil and enter the body after injury, often through a puncture wound, wounds contaminated by dirt or splinters, or wounds caused by burns. The wound may be trivial or unnoticed, such as a skin puncture caused by a rose thorn. Toxin from the anaerobic tetanus bacilli (*Clostridium tetani*) causes painful muscle spasms. Complications include:

- lockjaw
- painful muscular spasms
- death.

The five doses of tetanus between infancy and mid-teens, which children receive in the British schedule, probably give lifelong immunity; but a booster dose given for an injury, 10 or more years after the previous dose of vaccine, gives extra protection.

PERTUSSIS (WHOOPING COUGH)

In the early 1950s, the average annual number of cases of whooping cough reported was above 100 000, with a death rate of one in every

1000. In the 10 years after introduction of the pertussis vaccine in 1957, this number fell to fewer than 30 000. In 1974, when immunization rates were over 80%, only 10 000 cases were reported. However, in the same year Kulenkampff *et al.*[4] published the results of a study of 36 children admitted to hospital with severe neurological illness, 33 of whom had received pertussis vaccine during the week preceding onset of illness. The report referred to the possible risk factors associated with the vaccine, although the study did not include a control group. Widespread publicity of this report, which appeared to question the safety of pertussis vaccine, resulted in a dramatic decline in immunized children. Only three out of every ten children born in 1976 had been immunized against pertussis 2 years later. In consequence, two major epidemics of whooping cough occurred, the first in 1977–79, with over 100 000 cases and 36 deaths in the UK, and the second in 1982, with almost 66 000 cases and 14 deaths in England and Wales.[5]

The National Childhood Encephalopathy Study[6] examined carefully the reported cases of 'brain damage' in infants who had had pertussis and other vaccinations. The study concluded that there was no certain proof that pertussis vaccine had caused neurological damage, but if there was a risk it was probably about one in 300 000 vaccinations. As this risk, if it occurs at all, is much less than the risk of encephalopathy (brain injury) or death from whooping cough, the confidence in pertussis vaccine returned. The experience of whooping cough in other countries that stopped or reduced the use of pertussis vaccine, e.g. Germany and Japan, and trials of new acellular (purified) pertussis vaccines have confirmed the efficacy and safety of the whole-cell pertussis vaccine that is still in use in the UK today. Since 1979, immunization rates have risen to 94% of children by the age of 2 in 1997. As a consequence, whooping cough notifications have fallen to less than 5000 a year.

Whooping cough is caused by the highly communicable bacterium, *Bordetella pertussis,* which primarily affects the trachea and bronchi, resulting in episodes of paroxysmal coughing and vomiting, which can last for over 6 weeks. The child is infectious for 3 weeks unless an antibiotic, such as erythromycin, is given. This will not lessen the illness but is said to reduce the infectious period to 5 days.[7] A full course of vaccine (three doses) protects 80–90% of recipients. Complications include:

- convulsions

- pneumonia

▨ lung damage

▨ temporary and/or permanent brain damage

▨ subconjunctival haemorrhage

▨ death (especially in babies aged less than 6 months).

There has been a steady increase in the number of reported cases of pertussis since 1992, of which more than a quarter of cases were in people aged 15 years and over. Recent publications have highlighted the importance of pertussis in adults, where the clinical presentation is not distinctive and likely to be missed. The cohort of young adults born in the 1970s and early 1980s may not have been immunized, and if infected themselves are highly likely to infect their own babies. There is no upper age limit, and acellular pertussis vaccine should be offered to young adults who have not previously been vaccinated, and who have no history of whooping cough.

HAEMOPHILUS INFLUENZAE TYPE B (HIB)

In the past, one in every 600 children had Hib meningitis or epiglottitis before the age of 4 years. One in 20 of the children who had Hib meningitis died from the infection despite antibiotic treatment, and one in ten had deafness or other neurological damage. Epiglottitis is inflammation of the throat, which blocks the entrance to the windpipe. Children with this infection died by suffocation unless they were treated immediately by antibiotics, and in some cases, by a tracheostomy. Routine vaccination began in 1992, using a purified polysaccharide conjugated to a protein (e.g. tetanus toxoid). Since the introduction in 1992 of Hib vaccination as routine for all infants, with a catch-up programme for children up to the age of 4 years, the risk of disease has reduced to 2–3% of the incidence before 1992 in the UK. Vaccination against Hib not only protects the vaccinated child, but also reduces the spread of this bacterium. A similar benefit of protecting others in the family and community has been observed for whooping cough, measles and rubella.

HEPATITIS B

Hepatitis B is a blood-borne virus infection that is often asymptomatic in children who may acquire the infection at birth if their mothers are carriers, or under conditions of poor hygiene from other infected children, presumably by the contamination of cuts and skin sores. In adults, infection is typically sexually transmitted. In people of any age, it can be spread by contaminated needles or in unscreened blood transfusions. Infection in adults may present as acute hepatitis with jaundice and fever. Recovery is the usual outcome, although one in 1000 cases may have a fulminant infection. The main medical problem is the chronic infection that follows in about 10% of cases. This chronic infection can cause cirrhosis and liver cancer, and the carrier remains a potential source of infection to others. For these reasons, hepatitis B vaccines have been used firstly for high-risk groups, i.e. people who, because of their place of residence, work, sexual behaviour or drug-use, are more likely to become infected and to carry the hepatitis B virus. More recently, it has been realized that selective programmes may only prevent a fraction of the cases, and that a wider use would be more effective. Therefore many countries are introducing universal hepatitis B vaccination, either combined with the infant vaccines, or given to teenagers in school. Such programmes are expensive, although calculations show that the cost is not excessive when the benefits are compared with other medical treatments.

While a decision is awaited for a UK programme, it is important that the current recommendations for selective vaccination are applied. This includes:

- identifying women who are hepatitis B carriers in pregnancy and vaccinating their babies at birth

- siblings of children identified to be hepatitis B positive

- children who are brought up in residential institutions for people with learning disability.

POLIOMYELITIS

Poliovirus, of which there are three types (I, II and III), damages nerve cells. Man is its only natural host, carrying the virus in the intestine and spreading it by faecal contamination of hands, food or water. In the disease the virus is carried from the intestine to the brain and spinal cord. The virus inflames the linings of the brain (the meninges) and the nerves that carry impulses from the brain to the muscles. An epidemic can quickly occur in an unprotected community. Complications include:

- meningitis

- temporary or permanent paralysis, with lameness in mild cases and paralysed breathing muscles in severe cases

- death.

Routine vaccination began in 1956 in the UK using injected, inactivated poliomyelitis vaccine (IPV; Salk). This was replaced in 1962 with oral, live attenuated vaccine (OPV; Sabin). Notifications of paralytic poliomyelitis have dropped from nearly 4000 in 1955 to 257 in 1960. Between 1974 and 1978, 35 cases were reported. Since 1993 there has been an average of one case per year, of whom two out of three are vaccine-associated cases. Vaccine-associated cases are either infants or their unvaccinated relatives who have been infected by the live vaccine strain of virus. The poliomyelitis in these cases tends to be milder than the wild infection. These adverse events are very rare compared with the millions of doses of polio vaccine used, but they emphasize the reason for using an inactivated polio vaccine (IPV) for people who have immunodeficiency. A few of the cases of poliomyelitis in the UK are due to infection acquired abroad; and overseas travel to countries which have yet to control polio has been an indication for a booster dose.

   This reason for booster doses is becoming less applicable. In the American continent, a concerted vaccination programme has eliminated polio since 1994. Intense surveillance is in place to check that this happy state of affairs is true and maintained. Given the geographical, political and social problems that exist in some parts of the Americas, this achievement offers the hope of global eradication by the year 2000. Mass campaigns (e.g. National Immunization Days) towards this objective are being used in Asia and Africa.

MEASLES/MUMPS/RUBELLA (MMR)

Measles

Measles is highly contagious and is a notifiable disease. It is transmitted by droplet infection and is characterized by Koplik spots, rash, fever, coryza, conjunctivitis and bronchitis. Incubation is about 10 days, with a further 2–4 days before the rash appears. It is infectious from the beginning of the prodromal stage until 4 days after the appearance of the rash. Case fatality is age related, high in children under 1 year of age, lowest in children aged 1–9 years and rises with advancing age. Complications are reported in one in 15 notified cases and include:

- otitis media

- bronchitis

- pneumonia

- febrile convulsions

- encephalitis

- subacute sclerosing panencephalitis

- death.

Whilst the serious neurological complications are rare, encephalitis occurs in one in 5000 cases, with a mortality of 15%, and 20–40% suffering permanent neurological sequelae. Subacute sclerosing panencephalitis (SSPE) is extremely rare, but is a fatal late complication, often following early measles infection which may not have been recognized. Immunization protects against SSPE.

Until the introduction of measles vaccine in 1968 the average annual number of cases varied between 160 000 and 800 000. In 1968 there were 90 deaths from measles. By the mid-1970s the annual number of cases had dropped to 50 000–180 000. Between 1970 and 1988 an average of 13 children died each year from measles or its complications. This vaccine, which protected against measles alone, was safe and offered 95% protection, but the take-up was disappointingly low, with national immunization figures for single-antigen measles never exceeding 65%. The introduction of

MMR vaccine in October 1988, with uptake levels in excess of 90%, led to a dramatic decrease in measles notification. Since 1988 there have only been 11 deaths due to measles recorded in England and Wales. By 1993 there were less than 10 000 measles notifications a year, down to 3962 in 1997.

Because of high MMR coverage, transmission was greatly reduced amongst younger children. This resulted in a rising proportion of susceptible school-age children, and predictions of a major resurgence of measles amongst the school-age population. Measles epidemics had been demonstrated in many other countries following similar periods of low incidence achieved through high immunization coverage. In November 1994, over 8 000 000 children aged between 5 and 16 years were immunized throughout the UK in a mass campaign. Susceptibility in the target population has fallen sevenfold, and the few confirmed cases are mostly in adults or children too young to be immunized, and can often be linked to importation of the virus from abroad.

Mumps

Mumps is caused by a *Paramyxovirus*, transmitted by droplet spread from infected saliva. It causes swelling of the parotid glands, which may be unilateral or bilateral. The incubation period is between 14 and 21 days, with transmission from several days before the parotid swelling to several days after it appears. It was made a notifiable disease in October 1988, since when notifications have fallen progressively. Laboratory testing shows that most notified cases are not mumps. Complications include:

- meningitis
- encephalitis
- orchitis
- oophoritis
- sensorineural hearing loss
- pancreatitis.

Mumps vaccine was introduced because it was the commonest cause of viral meningitis in the under-15 age group, resulting in 1200 hospital admissions every year. **Even when orchitis is bilateral,**

there is no firm evidence of sterility. Orchitis was never the reason for introduction of mumps vaccine.

Rubella (German measles)

Rubella is a mild, infectious disease causing transient erythematous rash and lymphadenopathy involving post-auricular and sub-occipital glands. Rarely, in adults, it can cause arthritis and arthralgia.

If rubella is contracted during early pregnancy, especially during the first 8–10 weeks of gestation, it can result in fetal damage in up to 90% of cases, and multiple defects are common (congenital rubella syndrome). The risk of fetal damage declines to about 10–20% by 16 weeks and after then, is rare. The baby may be still-born or suffer from one or more of the following handicaps:

- blindness

- cataracts

- deafness (or impaired hearing)

- heart damage

- intrauterine growth retardation

- mental retardation

- inflammatory lesions of the brain, liver, lungs and bone marrow.

The rubella virus was identified in 1962 and live, attenuated rubella virus vaccine has been offered to schoolgirls aged 10–14 years and non-immune women since 1970. It induces an antibody response in 95% of those immunized and offers long-term protection.

The inclusion of rubella vaccine in 1988 with measles and mumps vaccines as MMR led to a considerable decline in rubella in young children. There has been a substantial increase in notifications and laboratory-confirmed cases amongst young adult males, who were not vaccinated in rubella immunization programmes. In addition was an increase in reported rubella infections in pregnant women, rising from two in 1992 to 25 in 1993, but declining to ten in 1995. The schoolgirl programme stopped after the mass measles–rubella campaign in 1994.

New recommendations

To prevent the re-emergence of epidemics of measles and rubella, a two-dose schedule of MMR was introduced in October 1996. The first dose is recommended shortly after the first birthday and a reinforcing dose before school entry. These should be given irrespective of a history of measles, mumps, or rubella infection. The second dose is intended to vaccinate the small proportion of children who have not responded fully to the first dose, and to offer a chance of vaccination to children who missed MMR vaccine when younger.

TUBERCULOSIS

Routine vaccination of schoolchildren with BCG vaccine against tuberculosis was introduced in the 1950s, although a marked decline in notifications and deaths from the disease was already occurring. The vaccine is 70–80% effective and gives protection for at least 15 years. The incidence of tuberculosis (TB) continued to decline, from 117 000 notifications of cases and almost 50 000 deaths in 1913, to about 6000 cases a year in the UK. Much of this improvement is due to better treatment and to better standards of living. It is estimated that the contribution that BCG vaccination makes to the control of TB is in the order of 100–200 fewer young adult cases a year. It had been expected that the national programme of BCG vaccination would cease to be needed by 1996, but the entrenchment of TB in inner cities and the emergence of multidrug-resistant TB have led to greater caution in stopping.

Tuberculosis is commonly caused by the organism *Mycobacterium tuberculosis,* and is acquired through airborne transmission from an infected person, often a member of the same household. Later complications may include:

■ infections of the lymph nodes

■ bronchiectasis and empyema

■ tuberculous meningitis

■ tuberculous peritonitis

■ tuberculous bones and joints

■ renal tuberculosis (rare).

The majority of health districts has continued to offer routine vaccination to all schoolchildren aged 10–14 years, who have been
shown to be tuberculin-negative following Mantoux or Heaf testing.
Some health districts, such as Oxfordshire, which discontinued
routine vaccination of schoolchildren and offered vaccination on a
selective basis, may resume the routine BCG programme in schools
because tuberculosis has not been adequately controlled in other
places. A few districts have offered BCG to all newborn children
because of a higher than normal incidence of tuberculosis in their
areas. Neonatal BCG policy is a key part of the WHO expanded
programme of immunization.

BCG is advisable for infants who:

■ are born to parents where either comes from a country with a
high rate of TB (see list). The reason for this is that the parent(s)
or grandparents may have had TB and that friends and relatives
from the high risk country may visit the family. Children are often
taken to visit the parents' family in high risk countries

or

■ will reside in or travel frequently to any area where the risk of TB
is high. This includes Caucasians going to developing countries
who have been born in this country

or

■ are living in the same house as 'old' cases of TB, however long
ago it occurred. This is because of the risk of TB reactivating. If
the infant is known to be a contact of a case of active TB he/she
should be referred to a paediatrician.

Skin colour does **not** always equate with high risk – it is the ethnicity
of the parents and the community that the infant belongs to which is
important. Babies born to 'white' families may also be at high risk,
e.g. families from Eastern Europe.

Countries with high rates of TB

Afghanistan; Albania; Algeria; Angola; Armenia; Azerbaijan
Bangladesh; Belize; Belorussia; Benin; Bhutan; Bolivia;
   Bosnia Herzegovina; Botswana; Brazil; Brunei; Bulgaria;
   Burkino Faso; Burundi
Cambodia; Cameroon; Cape Verde; Central African Republic;
   Chad; Comoros; Chile; China; Congo; Croatia
Djibouti; Dominican Republic
Ecuador; Egypt; El Salvador; Equatorial Guinea; Eritrea; Estonia;
   Ethiopia
French Guiana
Gabon; Gambia; Georgia; Ghana; Guinea; Guinea-Bissau
Haiti; Honduras; Hong Kong
India; Indonesia; Ivory Coast
Kazakhstan; Kenya; Korea; Kyrgyzstan
Laos; Latvia; Lesotho; Liberia; Libya; Lithuania
Macedonia; Madagascar; Malawi; Malaysia; Maldives; Mali;
   Mauritania; Mauritius; Moldova; Mongolia; Morocco;
   Mozambique; Myanmar (Burma)
Namibia; Nepal; Nicaragua; Niger; Nigeria
Pakistan; Papau New Guinea; Panama; Paraguay; Peru;
   Philippines; Poland
Réunion; Romania; Russian Federation; Rwanda
Saint Helena; São Tomé & Principe; Senegal; Sierra Leone;
   Singapore; Slovenia; Solomon Isles; Somalia; South Africa;
   Sri Lanka; Sudan; Swaziland
Taiwan; Tajikistan; Tanzania; Thailand; Togo; Tunisia; Turkey;
   Turkmenistan
Uganda; Ukraine; Uzbekistan
Vietnam
Yemen; Yugoslavia
Zaire; Zambia; Zimbabwe

These countries are those estimated by WHO as having an incidence of tuberculosis greater than 50 per 100 000. Some European
countries, e.g. Greece, Italy and Spain have an estimated incidence
approaching 50 per 100 000. Risk to babies from these countries
needs to be considered in the light of other factors.

   These babies should receive BCG vaccine intradermally or by
percutaneous multiple puncture, either in the maternity unit or at
home by the community midwife or health visitor. If this selective

BCG has not been given at birth, it can be given at the same time (into the skin of the upper arm at the insertion of the deltoid) as the first doses of diphtheria, tetanus, pertussis, Hib (given into the thigh) and polio vaccines at 2 months of age. A Heaf test before vaccination is not necessary for children under 3 months old.

BCG is also recommended for children who arrive in Britain from countries where tuberculosis is common and for those in household contact with tuberculosis. A Heaf test and examination for the scar of a previous BCG vaccination should be done first.

A Heaf test uses the Heaf 'gun' to produce a circle of six small punctures after tuberculin PPD (protein purified derivative) solution has been applied to a small area of skin surface, usually the inner forearm. The Heaf test is performed before vaccination and is read 3–10 days later by the school nurse, health visitor, or GP.

It is best to do a Heaf test a month or more away from giving a live virus vaccine.

Reading a Heaf test

We recommend that readers who are unfamiliar with Heaf tests and BCG vaccination technique should study the excellent diagrams on the inside back cover and on pp. 234–5 of the DoH guidance *Immunisation against infectious disease*.[3] The table summarizes appropriate action following a Heaf test.

Table 1: Heaf test outcomes

Result		Action
Negative:	Nothing to see, or 3 raised papules	Not immune, vaccinate with BCG if a child or a young adult
Positive:	Grade 1: 4+ raised papules	As above, as if negative
	Grade 2: raised red ring with joined papules	Refer for chest X-ray and medical opinion, unless BCG was previously given
	Grade 3: raised red lump	Refer for chest X-ray and medical opinion
	Grade 4: vesiculated red lump	Refer for chest X-ray and medical opinion

Note: individuals who are HIV-positive should *not* receive BCG vaccine.

3

Immunization schedules

Primary immunization

At birth:

- hepatitis B vaccine for children born to women who carry hepatitis B virus. If the mother is carrying the hepatitis B 'e' antigen, the baby should have, in addition, a single dose of hepatitis B immunoglobulin, which should be given in the opposite thigh at birth. Two more doses of vaccine are needed at age 1 month and 6 months. The paediatric dose of hepatitis B vaccine is half the adult dose: 10 mcg (0.5 ml) instead of 20 mcg (1 ml)

- BCG for some babies of immigrant families, and those in household contact with TB

2 months

polio + diphtheria/tetanus/pertussis + Hib

3 months

polio + diphtheria/tetanus/pertussis + Hib

4 months

polio + diphtheria/tetanus/pertussis + Hib

12–15 months

measles/mumps/rubella

Secondary immunization

4–5 years (preschool)

boosters of polio + diphtheria/tetanus + MMR
This is a chance to catch up primary immunization to any children
who have missed out on earlier vaccinations

Tertiary immunization

10–14 years

BCG

13–18 years

polio + Td, tetanus/diphtheria (adult low dose)

All children should be immunized even if they present outside the
recommended ages. No opportunity to immunize should be missed,
and there is no upper age limit for immunization, including pertussis.
MMR can be given to *any* individual regardless of age. Children
attending for their school-leaving immunizations should have their
immunization status checked, and be offered MMR if appropriate.

OTHER SCHEDULES

■ If the child has arrived from overseas and is staying in the UK,
change to national schedule.

■ If there is doubt about which, if any, immunizations have been given, start a complete immunization programme.

■ If the child is returning abroad within 1 year, keep to the schedule of the country of origin.

■ For children from countries where measles vaccine is given *before* the first birthday, re-immunization will be necessary.

DELAYS IN THE IMMUNIZATION PROGRAMME

If immunizations have been delayed or interrupted, they should be resumed but not repeated, allowing appropriate intervals between the remaining doses. The intervals between giving the immunizations are 3–4 weeks between each of the first three immunizations of polio + DTP + Hib.

Live vaccines may be given simultaneously at different sites, or if this is either not possible or unacceptable, then a 3-week interval should be allowed.

If the child is late starting the primary immunization course, and is aged 12 months or more, the priority is to give MMR first. Oral polio + DTPHib (one injection) can be given at the same time as MMR immunization, in separate injection sites in opposing limbs. If this schedule is adopted, the remaining immunizations will only be polio + DTP, as one injection of Hib over 12 months of age offers adequate immunity. Alternatively, if the choice is single injections, oral polio should be given with MMR, and DTPHib may be given as soon after as possible.

Recent studies have shown that Hib vaccines are interchangeable and a course need not be re-started if the original brand is not available.

All children should be immunized, apart from the very few exceptions outlined in Chapter 4. A decision not to immunize a child should no longer be the 'easier' choice for the professional involved, and it is important to realize that it is a serious matter to withhold protection. Specialist advice (from a consultant in communicable diseases control or a paediatrician with particular knowledge and interest in immunization) should always be sought in doubtful cases.

'Catch up' needs to be considered with the parents of those children delayed in receiving MMR because of vaccine scares. Starting playgroup or nursery school can be used as prompts. Certainly, the second MMR scheduled for the pre-school medical examination is going to be important in preventing outbreaks of measles and rubella.

4

Special considerations and contraindications

Always take specialist advice before deciding not to vaccinate a child.

CONSIDERATIONS WHEN THE CHILD IS UNWELL

If the child has an acute severe illness, especially with a fever (above 38°C), then consider delaying immunization. This is not because the immunization may cause harm, but the vaccine may not be fully effective and it is important to be able to recognize a reaction. Minor illnesses without a fever, particularly upper respiratory tract infections, coughs without other symptoms, and mild diarrhoea and vomiting (except with polio), are not reasons for delaying immunization.

If the child is taking a course of antibiotics, but has no acute symptoms, do *not* delay immunization.

REACTIONS TO VACCINATION

Immunization should not be carried out in any individual with a history of severe local or general reaction to a preceding dose as defined below, without specialist medical advice either from a consultant in communicable diseases or a paediatrician with specialist knowledge and interest in immunization.

All adverse reactions should be reported on a yellow card to the Committee on the Safety of Medicines.

Local

■ An extensive area of redness and swelling, indurated and involving most of the anterolateral surface of the thigh or a major part of the circumference of the upper arm.

Please note that severe local reactions can result from poor technique, such as injections that are not into muscle or with too fine a needle so that the vaccine is not dissipated over a wide enough area. Technique should be checked, and specialist opinion sought with a view to separating subsequent injections (e.g. DTP + Hib).

General

■ Fever equal to or greater than 39.5°C within 48 hours of vaccine.

■ Anaphylaxis: an immediate reaction characterized by facial swelling, wheezing (bronchospasm), stridor (laryngeal oedema), and collapse.

■ Prolonged unresponsiveness.

■ Prolonged inconsolable or high-pitched screaming for more than 4 hours.

■ Convulsions or encephalopathy within 72 hours.

Ask for specialist advice on which vaccines should be given in future. Do not say that the child should never have another vaccination unless you are very certain that the vaccine has caused the reaction.

PERTUSSIS

Vaccination against pertussis (whooping cough) has been surrounded by more misunderstanding than any other vaccine used in the last 50 years. The present advice about special considerations and contraindications is based on much more knowledge than at the time of the whooping cough scare, 20 years ago.

The only definite contraindication to pertussis vaccine is a general reaction, as defined above, to a previous dose of the vaccine. In this respect, pertussis is the same as other vaccines. A child with a generalized reaction after DTP should have the course of immunization completed with DT vaccine.

Special consideration is required for:

■ a baby with a neurological problem that is still evolving when the baby is due for DTP (i.e. is approaching 2 months of age). Seek advice from a paediatrician, who will probably advise deferring pertussis vaccination until the child's neurological condition is stable

■ a severe local reaction to a previous dose. The advice is likely to be about reducing local reactions by better technique, and by separating the DT, pertussis and Hib injections.

Parents' views should play an important part in these considerations. Pertussis vaccination is recommended for:

■ children with epilepsy or a history of convulsions

■ children with a family history of epilepsy

■ children who have had cerebral damage in the neonatal period

because neurological complications are considerably more common after whooping cough infection than after pertussis vaccination. Fits after DTP and DT are rarer when these vaccines are given before the age of 6 months, as in the UK schedule. This is because febrile convulsions are uncommon before this age. So there is no advantage in delaying vaccination. If in doubt, ask for a specialist medical opinion from a consultant community paediatrician, district immunization coordinator or consultant in communicable disease control, before proceeding with pertussis vaccination.

Specialist advice must be sought before deciding not to offer pertussis vaccination.

The following are *not* contraindications to pertussis vaccine:

▩ a family history of idiopathic epilepsy in first-degree relatives

▩ a family history of febrile convulsions

▩ idiopathic epilepsy in other than first-degree relatives

▩ asthma, eczema, hay fever, migraine, food allergy, other allergies in the child or child's family

▩ antibiotics

▩ chronic diseases, particularly heart and lung

▩ failure to thrive

▩ low birth weight and/or prematurity.

After vaccination, some babies have a spell of crying, apparently inconsolably. This is not specific to pertussis vaccines and it has no significance in long-term effects, but it may make parents reluctant for their child to have a second dose. The acellular pertussis vaccines are less likely to have this effect than the currently-used whole-cell vaccines, which is one reason why they have been developed. The drawback of the earlier acellular vaccines is that they give slightly less protection than the whole-cell vaccines used routinely in Europe (efficacy of 80–85% as opposed to 80–90%). The most recent assessment of pertussis vaccines studied in Sweden and Italy, found that the whole-cell vaccine used in the UK gave equal protection against whooping cough.[8] The best acellular pertussis vaccine had five components (antigens). Some of the three and two component vaccines were not quite so effective.

For parents who do not want their child to have the whole-cell pertussis vaccine, an acellular vaccine is available on a named patient basis (a named patient basis applies to unlicensed vaccines supplied for specified individuals). This should be given at the same time as DT, Hib and polio, if possible. If this is not possible, then the course of pertussis vaccine can be completed by giving the acellular vaccine on its own, so that the child receives a total of three doses of pertussis vaccine. When a course has been started with whole-cell vaccine, the course can be completed with acellular vaccine – there is no need to start the course again.

If a child coming for a pre-school vaccination has not had pertussis vaccine as an infant, vaccination should be offered. The regimen is:

1 pre-school booster of DT given as DTP (i.e. with whole-cell vaccine)

2 a month later, a dose of acellular pertussis vaccine

3 another month later, a second dose of acellular pertussis vaccine.

CONTRAINDICATIONS TO LIVE VACCINES

The live vaccines are:

- BCG
- MMR (measles, mumps, rubella)
- oral polio (OPV).

Children receiving high-dose corticosteroids (2 mg per kilo per day > a week)

Immunization with live vaccines should be postponed until 3 months after cessation of high-dose steroid treatment.

Children on immunosuppressive treatment, including general irradiation; malignancies such as lymphoma, leukaemia, Hodgkin's disease or other tumours of the reticuloendothelial system

Immunization with live vaccines should be postponed until 6 months after cessation of treatment.

Children with impaired immunological mechanisms, e.g. hypogammaglobulinaemia

If these children are in contact with measles or chickenpox they should receive immunoglobulin as soon as possible. Specialist advice should be taken on whether to give live vaccines after 3 months.

Siblings of children with contraindications

It is essential to ensure that siblings and close contacts – including adults – of children for whom live vaccines are contraindicated, have received their full immunization schedule. In the event of these individuals needing polio vaccine, IPV should be administered. There is *no* risk of contracting measles, mumps, rubella or TB from contact with a recently immunized individual.

Immunoglobulin

Injected live vaccines should not be administered within 3 months after an injection of immunoglobulin, because the antibodies in the immunoglobulin may stop the vaccine from working. This effect is unlikely to interfere with oral polio vaccine, if the baby had immunoglogulin for hepatitis B or neonatal varicella zoster at birth. If a live vaccine has been given within 3 months of immunoglobulin, the live vaccination can be repeated when the 3 months have passed.

MEASLES/MUMPS/RUBELLA

- MMR vaccine should not be given within 3 months of an injection of immunoglobulin.

- If the child has an acute febrile illness, immunization should be postponed until the child is recovered.

- If a child has untreated malignant disease or altered immunity, is receiving immunosuppressive or radiation treatment or high-dose systemic steroids, give vaccine 6 months after cessation of treatment.

- If a child has a history of allergy to neomycin or kanamycin (extremely rare) do not give MMR vaccine.

- If another live vaccine by injection has been given within 3 weeks, give vaccine after 3 weeks.

- If administered to adult women, pregnancy should be avoided for one month.

Egg allergy

Increasing evidence shows that MMR can be given safely to children even with previous history of anaphylaxis (generalized urticaria, swelling of the mouth and throat, difficulty in breathing, hypotension or shock) following food containing egg. Dislike of or refusal to eat eggs is not a contraindication. If there is concern, ask a consultant paediatrician to see the child with a view to vaccinating in hospital as a day case.[9]

Minor reactions which show that the vaccine has taken effect

- Because of the risk of the common, mild, febrile reaction to the measles component which can occur 5–10 days after the injection and last for 2–3 days, parents should be given advice about care of the feverish child. *Keep the child as cool as possible – plenty of cool drinks, remove clothing, tepid sponging – and administer junior paracetamol if appropriate.*

- Parotid swelling may occur 3 weeks after immunization.

- Children with either a febrile reaction or with parotid swelling are *not* infectious.

Children in the following categories are at particular risk from measles infection and *should* be immunized with MMR vaccine:

■ children with febrile convulsions or ordinary convulsions, or a close family history of idiopathic epilepsy

■ children with chronic conditions such as cystic fibrosis, congenital heart or kidney disease, Down's syndrome, failure to thrive

■ children over 1 year of age in residential or day care, including playgroups and nursery schools.

Children with a personal or family history of asthma, eczema, hay fever, migraine or food allergy, or taking antibiotics should be vaccinated. A history of measles, mumps or rubella, is *not* a contraindication, and there are no ill effects from vaccinating individuals who are already immune. In young children these diseases are often misdiagnosed since the diseases have become uncommon.

MMR can be used to protect susceptible individuals during a measles outbreak providing it is administered within 3 days of exposure, and should be given regardless of immune status. This does not apply to exposure to mumps or rubella, as the antibody response to these infections is too slow for effective prophylaxis.

It has been suggested that the measles virus is a cause of Crohn's disease – a chronic inflammation of the ileum and colon. This theory is only one of several explanations for Crohn's disease, and there is more reason for wanting to prevent measles by vaccination than for not giving measles vaccine because of this suggestion.

POLIOMYELITIS

The following are *not* contraindications for giving polio vaccine:

■ breast-feeding – this does not interfere with the vaccine, even if a feed is given soon after the vaccine

■ antibiotics – these do not interfere with the vaccine

■ if the baby vomits within 1 hour of receiving the vaccine – repeat the dose.

Faecal excretion may last up to 6 weeks and, rarely, may lead to infection of unimmunized contacts. Good personal hygiene should be advised for all contacts of recently-immunized babies – in particular, washing hands after nappy changes. Offer vaccine to un-immunized relatives, e.g. grandparents, by a course of three doses of oral polio vaccine at intervals of 4 weeks at the same time as the baby; there is no need to boost previously-immunized individuals.

Children for whom a live vaccine is contraindicated

Inactivated polio vaccine (IPV) should be given to children for whom a live vaccine is contraindicated, such as those with immuno-suppression from disease or therapy. IPV should also be used for siblings and household contacts, if appropriate.

HIV-POSITIVE CHILDREN

HIV-positive children, with or without symptoms, should receive all vaccines, *except* BCG vaccine. No harmful effects have been reported following immunization with live attenuated vaccines for measles, mumps, rubella and polio in HIV-positive children, who are at increased risk from these diseases.

IPV should be used instead of OPV for HIV-positive children, as excretion of the vaccine virus in the faeces may continue for longer than 6 weeks. Strict personal hygiene should be advised, emphasizing careful hand-washing at each nappy change.

5

Immunization procedure

SUITABILITY FOR IMMUNIZATION

Before the first course of immunization is given, the child must have been seen by a doctor and found to be suitable for immunization. A prescription must then be signed by the doctor in the personal child health record (PCHR) or other document. This prescription can act for the whole of the primary course of immunizations. Verbal authorization may be acceptable in special situations as long as the prescription is subsequently signed by the authorizing doctor.

Before each immunization the health of the child should be assessed by the person giving the injection by:

- asking if the child is well

- asking whether there were any adverse reactions to the previous dose

- checking that there have been no changes in the parents' decision.

Minor coughs or colds or being on a course of antibiotics should not postpone immunization, but a feverish, acutely unwell child should not be immunized that day. There is no evidence that immunizing an acutely unwell child is harmful, but it is less easy to differentiate between a possible reaction to the vaccine and the signs of the acute illness.

REACTIONS TO PREVIOUS IMMUNIZATIONS

A severe reaction, as defined in the previous chapter, to a previous dose of vaccine is the only absolute contraindication for omitting subsequent doses of, for example, pertussis vaccine. The future immunization schedule for such a child should be discussed with a consultant in communicable diseases or with a paediatrician with specialist knowledge and interest in immunization.

If there has been any reaction other than a severe local or general reaction, the child should continue with the planned immunization schedule, but where there is concern seek specialist advice.

ILLNESS SINCE THE LAST IMMUNIZATION

If the child has developed fits or had any serious illness or neurological symptoms since the last immunization, seek appropriate advice from the GP, consultant paediatrician or consultant in communicable disease control.

IMMUNIZATION CLINICS[10]

■ Clinics should be held at regular times on fixed days.

■ Surgeries should have a well-advertised commitment to opportunistic immunization, and parents should be encouraged to use this service if necessary.

■ Consideration should be given to those parents collecting siblings from playgroups, nurseries, school etc. when planning clinic times.

■ Opportunistic immunization should be offered whenever an unimmunized child attends surgery, even if only accompanying a parent.

▓ Immunization clinics should be linked to 'health visitor only' clinics.

▓ Interpreters or liaison workers should be available for families where English is not the first language.

INFORMATION FOR PARENTS

It is essential that parents receive correct advice. The Patient's Charter states that all individuals have the right '. . . *to be given a clear explanation of any treatment proposed, including any risks and alternatives, before deciding whether to agree to that treatment'.* Health workers must be up-to-date with recent changes and re-commendations, and check that their colleagues are also aware of any changes. The DoH guide, *Immunisation against infectious disease,*[3] is packed with useful information. If a question from a parent raises uncertainties, seek the correct answer *before* giving an immunization.

Health professionals are responsible for ensuring that parents receive accurate and consistent information in order that they may make an informed decision about immunization. This information comes largely from the DoH and its agents like the Health Education Authority. As such, the information is sometimes criticized as being one-sided, dealing only with the positive reasons for immunization and not considering parents' fears and the hazards of immunization. Whilst this point is acknowledged, we also know that the DoH gets its advice from doctors, nurses and scientists who have both con-siderable expertise and professional independence. These expert advisers are bound to put the interests of children's health ahead of all other considerations.

It may be a measure of the success of vaccination that there are some opponents who write and speak about disadvantages of vaccination in the UK. This group is well-read in the expand-ing body of non-medical literature on the subject which emanates from the UK, USA and Australia. This information is contained in books, articles and newsletters as well as television and video, and health professionals advising on immunization must be aware of it.

Since these opponents of vaccination may be quoted by parents when vaccinations are discussed, a list of some documents is given below:

What doctors don't tell you. L McTaggart. Wallace Press. 1993

Vaccination and immunisation: dangers, delusions and alternatives (what every parent should know). L Chaitow. CW Daniel Co. Ltd. 1990

A Shot in the Dark. HL Coulter and BL Fisher. Avery Publishing Group, Inc. 1991

Vaccination, social violence and criminality: the medical assault on the American brain. HL Coulter. North Atlantic Books. 1990

Immunization: the reality behind the myth. Walene James. Bergin and Garvet. 1988

Rubella vaccination: a failure. M Nightingale. *EPoCH* **5** (1): 3–4. 1982

Vaccination: a sacrament of modern medicine. R Moskowitz. *The Homeopath* **12** (1): 124–41. 1992

The hand that rocks the cradle. Health Care Reform Group. 1992.

CONSENT

■ Immunization requires informed consent. Therefore all health professionals involved with immunization must ensure that parents are informed:
  – that it is proposed to immunize the child
  – which immunization(s) are to be given
  – what protection they offer
  – what side-effects are common and what are the risks
  – any rare, severe side-effects.

■ In many places, appointments for immunization are sent by computer systems. In such systems, there may be forms for parents to sign well before the day when the child is brought for immunization. This consent is *only* for the child to be included in the immunization programme. In other systems, such consent is assumed for all children born in the district. In either case, be sensitive to parents' wishes that some immunizations are not given.

▪ Consent may be written or verbal. Written consent is self-evident, but verbal consent is adequate if it is witnessed.

▪ Seek consent, expressed verbally or in writing, each time a child is brought for immunization, after assessing the child's fitness and suitability.

▪ Consent is clearly implied when a parent brings the child for the immunization, exposes the injection site on request and allows the injection to be given.

▪ If every effort has been made to inform parents of immunization sessions in school, attendance of the child at school on the day may be viewed as acceptance that the child may be immunized, provided that there are no reservations expressed to the contrary.

▪ A child under 16 years of age may give consent for immunization, provided she or he fully understands the benefits and risks involved. However, she or he should be encouraged to involve a parent or guardian in this decision, if possible. Equally, respect the wishes of a child under 16 years of age who understands the benefits and risks, and refuses to be immunized.

▪ Children in care may need the written consent of Social Services if parental consent has not been given.

IMMUNIZATION BY NURSES

The DoH 1996 recommendations for immunization[3] say that a doctor may delegate responsibility for immunization to a nurse, provided the following conditions are fulfilled:

1 the nurse is willing to be professionally accountable for this work

2 the nurse has received training and is competent in all aspects of immunization, including the contraindications to specific vaccines

3 adequate training has been given in the recognition and treatment of anaphylaxis.

If these conditions are fulfilled and nurses carry out the immunization in accordance with the policies of the District Health Authority, NHS Trust or Health Board, the Authority/Trust/Board will accept responsibility for this. Similarly, nurses employed by general practitioners should have protocols for the above conditions.

Immunization by nurses without a doctor being present is a proactive response to those few children for whom it is difficult to be immunized through the conventional route, i.e. immunization clinics. With agreed protocols, practice nurses should be able to offer opportunistic immunization for those children presenting at surgeries outside the usual time. Similarly, health visitors are in a prime position to offer domiciliary and/or opportunistic immunization either in the home or other venue, such as clinic or playgroup.

OPPORTUNISTIC AND DOMICILIARY IMMUNIZATIONS

Opportunistic immunizations are those given when a child attends a doctor or nurse for some other purpose. They, and immunization at the child's home, are worthwhile options for some children. There will always be a minority of children who consistently fail to attend for their scheduled immunizations. The reasons for non-attendance may be because of inaccessibility of the clinic, inconvenient clinic times, chronic illness (either in the child or family) and very mobile families, such as those living in bed and breakfast and traveller gypsies. Health professionals should be non-judgemental in their approach to these families and should not refuse to consider opportunistic or domiciliary immunization because of their own preconceived ideas. For example, middle class families may often be considered 'well able' to get their child to the clinic because they have a car, and some families may be labelled as not caring sufficiently to bring their child.

Any child who either falls behind on the immunization schedule, or consistently fails to attend child health clinics should be considered a priority for opportunistic or domiciliary immunization, irrespective of the perceived individual circumstances.

TECHNIQUE AND ADMINISTRATION

With the exception of OPV and BCG, immunizations should be given by intramuscular or deep subcutaneous injection into the antero-lateral aspect of the thigh. They should never be given in the buttock because of the risk of sciatic nerve damage and also because of reduced efficacy of immunization when administered into adipose tissue. BCG is always administered intradermally or percutaneously, and never subcutaneously or intramuscularly. BCG is probably best given in the skin of the upper arm, over the insertion of the deltoid muscle. This site is clean and easily inspected during checks for immunity to tuberculosis.

We recommend that the needle size should be a 23 G (blue), apart from intradermal BCG, because this ensures that the injection is intramuscular or deep subcutaneous. The wider bore needle allows the vaccine to dissipate over a wider space, thus reducing the risk of localized redness and swelling.

Table 2: Administration of vaccines

Vaccine	Route of administration	Dose	Needle size
OPV	Oral	3 drops	Not relevant
IPV	Deep subcutaneous or intramuscular	0.5 ml	23 G
DTP, DT, Hib	Intramuscular *	0.5 ml	23 G
Measles/mumps/ rubella	Deep subcutaneous or intramuscular	0.5 ml	23 G
BCG	**Intradermal**	0.1 ml **Infants: 0.05 ml**	25 G
Hepatitis B	Intramuscular*	0.5 ml over 12 years: 1 ml	23 G

OPV – oral polio vaccine   DTP – diphtheria/tetanus/pertussis
IPV – inactivated polio vaccine   Hib – *Haemophilus influenzae* type b

* The authors believe that DTP causes less local reaction if given into muscle and not into the deep subcutaneous layer. Hepatitis B vaccine works better if given into muscle than when given into fat.

PROCEDURE

■ At the beginning of each session check expiry dates on the vaccines and adrenaline, and that storage conditions have been satisfactory.

■ Place adequate vaccine for the session in a rigid cool box with ice packs. *Never* work directly from the refrigerator.

■ Reconstituted vaccines must be used within the recommended period of reconstitution, 1–4 hours according to manufacturers' instructions. At the end of each immunization session all opened, unused vaccine should be discarded. Out-of-date, unused, spent or partly-used vials should be disposed of in sharps containers, for incineration.

■ Ensure adequate supplies of suitable syringes, needles, sharps disposal containers and relevant forms.

■ Ensure that *each* vaccinator has an anaphylaxis pack available.

■ Check that there have been no changes in the child's health, no adverse reactions to a previous dose and no changes in the consent.

■ Explain to parents which vaccine is to be given and the possibility of side-effects.

■ Check the dose and name of the vaccine and draw it up immediately before administering it. *Do not draw vaccine up for a session.*

■ Skin cleansing is not necessary for socially clean skin, and soap and water is an effective cleanser if necessary. However, if the injection site is cleansed with an alcohol-based swab, the skin should be dry before giving the immunization, as alcohol can inactivate live vaccine preparations.

■ The preferred injection site for babies is the anterolateral aspect of the thigh, and for older children, the deltoid muscle, using an appropriate needle for an adequate deep subcutaneous or intramuscular injection (23 G).

■ The exception to this is for BCG vaccine, which is *always* given intradermally, over the insertion of the left deltoid muscles using a 25 G needle. The skin should be stretched between the thumb and forefinger of one hand, and the needle inserted with the other, bevel upwards, for about 2 mm, almost parallel with the skin surface. A raised, blanched bleb will appear. For the Mantoux or Heaf test, the intradermal injection site is the middle of the flexor of the forearm.

- Dispose of syringe and needle into a rigid sharps container. *Do not resheath needles.*

- Complete the PCHR and relevant forms for data collection.

- Discard opened but unused vaccines at the end of each session. Single-dose vaccines can be ordered if necessary, for example, for a home immunization.

- Any unused vaccine in multidose containers which have been opened *must* be discarded at the end of each session.

RECORDING

It is very important that all immunizations are recorded and dated, both in the PCHR or other record for the parent, GP records, practice computer and child health system. If there are any enquiries or difficulties on this or other matters, contact (fill in your local names and numbers):

Post   *Name and telephone*

District Immunization Co-ordinator   _____

CCDC (if not the above)   _____

Child health computer manager   _____

Paediatricians with a special interest   _____

6

The care of vaccines

Vaccines are biological products and are susceptible to fluctuations in temperature. Manufacturers' instructions for storage and reconstitution of vaccines must be observed.

▨ Ordering and safe storage should be the responsibility of a suitably trained person, who is professionally accountable for this work, with a designated deputy to cover in times of absence.

▨ Childhood vaccines are free of charge and delivered to GP surgeries in England and Wales direct from the wholesalers, in refrigerated vans, either fortnightly or weekly. There should be no need to send vaccines by post.

▨ Vaccines should be refrigerated immediately on receipt, under correct storage conditions of between 0 and 4°C.

▨ Vaccines should *not* be stockpiled because of their sensitivity to incorrect storage.

▨ Vaccines should be stored so that the oldest is used first.

▨ Vaccines must not be exposed to direct sunlight or placed near sources of heat, such as radiators.

VACCINE REFRIGERATORS

- Refrigerators should be lockable in accordance with the Control of Substances Hazardous to Health (COSHH) Regulations 1988.

- Medical refrigerators are generally of a higher specification than domestic varieties, usually incorporating a fan and lock.

- Details of refrigerators and maximum/minimum thermometer suppliers may be obtained from the Communicable Disease Branch, DoH, Area 708, Wellington House, 133–155 Waterloo Road, London SE1 8UG (Tel: 0171 972 4472), or the Pharmaceutical Division, Scottish Office, DoH, St Andrew's House, Edinburgh EH1 3DE.

- If domestic refrigerators are used, the vaccines must be stored in the body of the fridge, never in the door.

- OPV should be stored at the bottom of the refrigerator where it is coolest.

- Vaccines should not be packed too tightly, and should never come into contact with ice in the refrigerator.

- Vaccines (or any other drugs) should never be stored in a refrigerator with foodstuffs.

REFRIGERATOR MAINTENANCE

- Stop the electricity supply from being inadvertently switched off by taping over the plug or switch and by placing a sign above the socket.

- Refrigerators should be checked annually by a qualified electrician and a written record should be kept.

- Refrigerators should be kept clean and defrosted according to the manufacturers' instructions.

- Vaccines should be stored with the maximum/minimum thermometer in another refrigerator or in a rigid cool box with ice packs during cleaning/defrosting.

TEMPERATURE CONTROL

▦ A maximum/minimum thermometer from a reputable supplier should be kept in the body of the refrigerator, irrespective of whether there is a temperature dial on the outside.

▦ Vaccines must never be stored below 0°C because of the risk of freezing which can cause deterioration of the vaccine as well as breaking the container.

▦ The maximum and minimum temperatures should be recorded regularly and at least at the beginning of each immunization session. The recorded readings should be documented, and the information kept for *21 years* in case of suspected vaccine failure.

▦ Special attention should be paid to the 'cold chain'. This concept is that all vaccines are kept at the correct temperature at all stages of transport and storage within the district. We recommend that each practice and each health district audits its cold chain regularly.

7

Reactions to immunization

Severe reactions are *rare* but it is important to be aware of the possibility and ensure that parents are aware of the risks and what should alert them. Listed below are the types of reaction which may occasionally occur, and the recommended actions.

MILD REACTIONS

About 15% of babies have a mild reaction to immunization in the first 48 hours following injection, with either some redness and soreness around the injection site or a slight fever and irritability. These mild reactions are not contraindications for further immunization. Parents should be warned of the possibility of such a reaction and given advice on managing a fever.

MANAGING A FEVER

Some babies develop a fever following immunization, and parents should be given advice on how to manage it.

■ Keep the baby as cool as possible – remove clothing; plenty of cool drinks, tepid sponging.

■ Junior paracetamol solution 2.5 ml (60 mg) for a child aged 2 months

■ Seek medical help if necessary.

IMMEDIATE REACTIONS

After any injection, or other medical procedure, a person may 'faint' or 'collapse'. The exact cause of the collapse is frequently hard to ascertain as there are difficulties in differentiating between breath-holding, vasovagal attacks (a faint) and anaphylactic reactions. Anaphylaxis is a theoretical risk with any vaccine, but a very thorough review by the Institute of Medicine[11] concluded that death due to anaphylaxis is extraordinarily rare: tetanus vaccine has the most reported life-threatening anaphylactic reactions, but the total is only 13 (only two fatal) cases – 11 adults and two children – despite billions of doses used in the last 60 years.

If a child collapses and then rapidly recovers, this is probably a vasovagal or breath-holding attack, and can be confirmed by the presence of peripheral pulses. Anaphylaxis, however, is determined by the following signs and symptoms:

■ pallor, limpness and apnoea

■ upper airway obstruction; hoarseness and stridor

■ lower airway obstruction; dyspnoea and wheezing

■ tachycardia and hypotension

■ bradycardia

■ urticaria.

MANAGEMENT OF A COLLAPSED PATIENT

■ Do not leave the child but ask a responsible person to dial 999 and summon medical aid.

▥ Place the child in the recovery position, insert an airway *only* if the patient is unconscious and if there has been proper training.

▥ In the absence of a strong central pulse, administer adrenaline 1:1000 by intramuscular injection, slowly, at a different injection site.

▥ If appropriate, begin cardiopulmonary resuscitation (CPR) until trained help arrives.

▥ If there is no improvement in 10 minutes, repeat the dose of adrenaline, up to a maximum of three doses.

Table 3: Recommended adrenaline doses in anaphylactic reactions

Age (years)	Dose (ml)
< 1	0.05
1	0.1
2	0.2
3–4	0.3
5	0.4
6–10	0.5
11–16	0.7
Adults	1.0 depending on build

▥ Intravenous (IV) chlorpheniramine maleate (Piriton) 2.5–5 mg may be given by *appropriately trained* individuals. IV hydrocortisone (100 mg) may also be given to prevent further deterioration.

▥ All cases should be admitted to hospital for observation.

▥ Report the reaction to the Committee on Safety of Medicines using the yellow card found in the back of the *British National Formulary* (BNF).

There is no good evidence for a policy of asking people to wait in the clinic for 20 minutes following an immunization. Recipients of vaccine should remain under observation until they have been seen to be in good health and not experiencing an immediate adverse reaction.

The local and general reactions that may occur with any vaccine are described on p. 28 of Chapter 4.

SPECIFIC REACTIONS

Pertussis immunization

Pollock *et al.*[12] in a study of the North West Thames region found that a neurological reaction, such as prolonged febrile convulsion, may occur in approximately one in 100 000 children receiving a full course of DTP, with almost none of these suffering a long-term effect. The Loveday case judgment rejected the *brain damage–pertussis vaccine* link.[13]

MMR immunization

Following the first dose of MMR, malaise, fever and/or a rash may occur, most commonly 7–10 days after injection, and usually lasting 24–48 hours. Febrile convulsions occur in one in 1000 children. Parotid swelling occurs in about 1% of children of all ages up to 4 years, usually 3 weeks after vaccination, although occasionally later. Febrile convulsions may occur, particularly if there is a simultaneous intercurrent infection, but the incidence is 8–10 times less than with the measles disease itself. Parents should be informed about the possibility of reactions, offered advice on the management of a fever (see p. 51) and reassured that the vaccine viruses are not transmitted to contacts.

In theory there is a risk of encephalitis or encephalopathy following MMR. However, a recent review of published evidence concluded that if there is a risk, it is exceptionally small.

After a second dose of MMR vaccine, adverse reactions are much less common, with studies showing no increase in fever or rash. Following the mass measles–rubella campaign in the Autumn of 1994, only three cases of thrombocytopenia were reported. Although the press reported that there were neurological complications, the three cases of Guillain–Barré syndrome that occurred in vaccinated children were well within the usual incidence of this syndrome that would be expected if there had not been this campaign.

Rubella immunization

Between 3 and 10% of girls may experience a mild reaction 1–3 weeks after rubella immunization, which may include fever, sore throat, rashes and joint pains.

DTP and Hib immunization

Local reactions from DTP and Hib injections are usually a sign that the injection was not given deeply enough, or that the patient has some existing immunity to one of the components (tetanus or diphtheria in particular). Check the technique of giving vaccines, especially that the needle is inserted to a depth of more than 2 cm (nearly an inch). In infants under 3 months of age, the mother's immunity to tetanus may have been carried over to the baby, in which case a lesser reaction can be expected from subsequent injections. In older children, it is worth checking the records to see whether the child has had an extra booster of tetanus after an injury.

8

Common worries

The child has a history of fits
Consult a specialist paediatrician before giving pertussis or measles vaccination but no matter what type of fit, it is completely safe to give polio, diphtheria, tetanus, BCG and rubella immunizations.

A relative, other than the parents or siblings has had fits
It is safe to give all immunizations, including pertussis and measles.

The baby had neonatal problems, and was in the Special Care Baby Unit
Most of these babies should be vaccinated against whooping cough, and for many the decision will have been taken by the time of discharge from the maternity unit and recorded in the discharge summary. If no decision has been taken, consult a specialist paediatrician about giving pertussis vaccine. It is safe to give all other immunizations.

The baby has had fits or is developing neurological problems
Refer to a specialist paediatrician for a decision about pertussis. It is safe to give all other immunizations.

The baby, or a relative, has asthma, eczema, hay fever or other allergies
It is safe to give all immunizations, including pertussis.

The baby has a rash
Mild eczema, nappy or heat rashes should not delay immunization.

The baby has a long-term chest or heart condition, such as cystic fibrosis or congenital heart disease

Chronically-ill babies are more susceptible to infections and should be immunized in accordance with the national schedule. However, as with all children, immunization should be postponed if the child is acutely unwell. Consideration should be given to immunizing these children at home when they are well to alleviate some of the extra burden experienced by the families.

The baby has been in contact with an infectious illness recently

If the baby is well, immunize. In some instances, such as measles infection, the immunization, if given in time, can stop the disease developing.

The baby is being given antibiotics

If the acute phase of the illness is over, it is safe to immunize. Antibiotics do not affect the immunization.

The mother is breast-feeding

Immunize. Breast-feeding is not a contraindication to immunization.

The baby was premature. When should immunizations start?

Immunizations should start 8 weeks after the baby was born, no matter how premature.

The baby weighs under 10 lb or 4.35 kg

Immunize 8 weeks after birth, whatever the weight. *The smaller the baby the greater the risk if the baby catches whooping cough.*

The child is aged over 2 years

Give any immunizations missed, including pertussis.

The child is aged over 10 years

Give any immunizations missed – there is no upper age limit to being immunized, including whooping cough (pertussis). Check whether any tetanus has already been given in casualty or by the GP. Use low (adult) dose diphtheria vaccine.

The immunization programme has been interrupted

There is no need to start the course again. The remaining doses should be given as if there had been no break, but if the child is aged over 13 months start with MMR.

Giving two immunizations at once

Two live vaccines can be given simultaneously (in different injection sites) or leave a 3-week gap between the two.
The live vaccines are:

- measles

- mumps

- rubella

- MMR

- polio.

BCG, also a live vaccine, *is the exception,* and should be given alone, with an interval of 3 weeks before giving another injected live vaccine.

The mother is pregnant

Immunizing the child will not affect the mother. It is safe to give any immunization to the child, and the mother may be better protected by having an immunized child.

The baby vomits after immunization

This is only important following polio, and only then if the baby vomits within the first hour. If this happens, repeat the dose as soon as possible on the same or next day.

Children who have recently entered the country with no immunization records

Try to find out what immunizations have been given. If in doubt treat as if unimmunized and start a complete programme. If the child is over 10 years old, use the low adult dose of diphtheria vaccine.

What about hepatitis B vaccine for children who are going to be exposed to hepatitis B and have not been vaccinated at birth?

The recognized reasons are hepatitis B in siblings, residential care for learning disability, and prolonged travel to a country of high endemicity.

RUBELLA

A child who has already had rubella
Immunize, since rubella is often misdiagnosed. There is no harm in immunizing twice.

A girl who may be pregnant
Do not immunize, but arrange for a rubella antibody test as part of the antenatal care. If antibody-negative, arrange for vaccination immediately after the baby is born. If the girl is not, after all, pregnant, arrange for contraceptive advice and vaccination together.

Women who have missed rubella vaccination at school
Women who went to school in countries where there has not been a rubella immunization programme, or for other reasons have missed vaccination, are susceptible to rubella transmitted from children and men. No opportunity should be missed to immunize young women of child-bearing age who have recently come to Britain.

A woman teacher who asks to be immunized against rubella
She should consult her GP and be given a blood test to check if she is already immune. If she has no immunity, she can be immunized if she is not pregnant and if she avoids becoming pregnant for 4 weeks following immunization.

IMMUNIZATION AND THE MEDIA

Concerns about adverse reactions to vaccination have been the subject of media attention since the discovery by Edward Jenner in 1796 that inoculating an individual with cowpox rendered them immune to smallpox. Cartoons were published depicting people growing cow-like parts.

The modern media offers greater coverage to health related issues and is far more sophisticated and influential. The public undoubtedly derives much information from various media sources, such as:

- newspapers

- television

- radio

- magazines – especially those aimed specifically at women and
  their children

- the Internet.

MMR

Since the introduction of MMR into the national schedule in 1988,
it has been an extremely popular vaccine – despite the overnight
withdrawal of two brands in 1992, following the identification of a
higher than expected risk of vaccine related aseptic meninigitis
linked to the Urabe strain of mumps virus used in their manufacture.

Contrary to popular media suggestion, measles is not a minor
childhood disease but a potential killer. Misinterpretation of recent
research has led to concern about the vaccine with a reported drop
of 1% in uptake of MMR. Continued concern could result in further
drops which would inevitably mean a recurrence of measles epidemics with possible deaths and considerable morbidity.

There are three important areas where concerns about MMR
have been raised.

MMR and Crohn's disease

Initial research published in 1993 suggested a causal link between
measles *infection* and Crohn's disease. However, subsequent research published in 1995 suggested that individuals immunized with
measles vaccine were three times more likely to develop Crohn's
disease.

This research was criticised for several reasons:

- the selection of the groups studied may have led to bias in that
  they differed in age and geographical location

- the hypothesis had not been tested vigorously enough to either
  be accepted or rejected

■ *all* subsequent research has found no link between measles vaccine and inflammatory bowel disease.

MMR and autism

This claim of a causal link between MMR and autism was first made in early 1997 and prompted a quick response from the National Autistic Society stating that:

'The updated prevalence information takes account of increased knowledge about the wide range of abilities of people with autism. . . These new figures do not indicate there is an increase in autistic disorders, but rather reflects an increased recognition of the range of the condition.'

There is also unpublished data to suggest that a rise in autism started over a decade before the introduction of MMR (Unpublished data, M Bax, D Lawton, Family Fund Trust).

The diagnosis of autism is often made around the time of MMR vaccination, with the temptation to misinterpret a temporal link as causal – as has happened with the most recent research. However, evidence to disprove this allegation from Sweden and the experience from the USA where MMR has been used for more than 25 years, with an excess of 250 million doses given worldwide, is often not mentioned by the media.

'MMR should be given as separate components'

This proposal has been suggested in the most recent research, and the argument has been encouraged by misinterpretation of the reasons why Japan currently offers MMR as separate injections. The Japanese experience is similar to that of the UK in 1992, with cases of post-vaccination aseptic meningitis linked to particular strains of mumps virus used in the manufacture. As in the UK, MMR vaccine was withdrawn but in the absence of an alternative licensed vaccine, measles, mumps and rubella have continued to be given as separate components.

Giving the vaccines as separate components would inevitably lead to poorer coverage of all three antigens and put unprotected children and their contacts at potential risk of serious disease.

The Chief Medical Officer, the JCVI and independent experts have been in consultation and have reviewed the published research and determined that there is no scientific research to prove a link between MMR and either inflammatory bowel disease or autism. This decision has been supported by the Assistant Director General of the WHO, Dr Ralph Henderson.

MMR remains the only safe and sensible method to protect not just our children, but the community as a whole.

9

Comments parents may make

This immunization business isn't necessary because the diseases were on the decline before vaccinations were invented

It is true that infectious diseases had become less common due to improved sanitation, housing, nutrition and safer water supplies. However, if you compare children who are immunized with children who are not, there will be more cases of disease in the unimmunized, and the few cases in the immunized group will be less severe.

There aren't many of these illnesses about these days

This is true, but nevertheless it is only because of effective immunization programmes that this is the case. While it is possible to eradicate some of the diseases – e.g. measles, mumps, rubella and polio – as has already been done with smallpox, this will not be possible without a good uptake of immunization. In the meantime, unless your child is adequately protected, s/he is still at risk.

Only poor children catch these illnesses – they're more common in Third World countries

It is true that these illnesses are more common and more severe in poorer countries where children are not as well-nourished. However, the infections can affect *any* child who is not immunized. There was a recent polio epidemic in a religious community in The Netherlands who had refused immunization. Despite their being well-fed and with good sanitation, one child died. In the rest of the surrounding population, all of whom were immunized, there were no cases. In addition, in the USA there have been problems with outbreaks of measles, whooping cough and rubella amongst religious communities that have refused immunization.

I'm going to keep my baby away from other children so s/he won't catch the germs

This will not work, because adults too can carry the germs, and sooner or later your child will meet other people. In addition, it is important to remember that tetanus can only be caught from spores in the soil, and you cannot protect your child from minor cuts or grazes which could result in tetanus.

They can treat all these illnesses these days

Some of the illnesses, such as whooping cough, diphtheria and Hib can be treated with antibiotics, but too often death or permanent disability occurs before treatment can be started. In the case of whooping cough, antibiotics only prevent the child being infectious, and in no way alleviate the length of the illness. Similarly, whilst antibiotics prevent diphtheria being infectious, they cannot prevent the toxin which is produced and which may cause permanent damage to the heart muscle, central nervous system and adrenal tissue. Whilst Hib can be treated with antibiotics, the treatment is only effective if the meningitis or epiglottitis is diagnosed and treatment started quickly. For the other infections for which we immunize, the only treatments are for the complications, not for the underlying disease.

My child is a year old; even if he gets one of these illnesses it won't affect him much

The illnesses may be serious whatever the age. Although whooping cough tends to be less serious the older it is caught, it may be transmitted to a small, vulnerable baby. Tetanus, diphtheria and polio are very serious whatever age they are contracted and measles tends to be more serious the older the individual. Rubella, whilst generally being a mild illness to the sufferer, can still cause catastrophic effects on the fetus. Mumps used to be the commonest cause of viral meningitis in the under 15s, and may also cause permanent unilateral deafness at any age.

I'm giving my child the homeopathic remedies. My homeopath says you shouldn't have orthodox vaccinations

There is no sound evidence that this is effective, and it is a common misconception that homeopaths condemn vaccination. The Faculty of Homeopathy, in fact, states quite clearly that all children should be immunized using the conventional vaccinations. An editorial in their journal in 1990 was quite categorical.

'Risk notwithstanding, to call for the abandonment of mass immunization would be criminally irresponsible, resulting, as it certainly would, in millions of unnecessary deaths. The anti-vaccination lobby has the right to argue its case, but must not be permitted to hitch its wagon to homeopathy's rising star. We are in danger of breeding a generation of spoilt brats, who think that, just because they have never seen a case of polio or diphtheria, the diseases never really existed.

Of course, the real reason they have not seen a case is precisely that mass immunization has been extremely successful. Hahnemann (the founder of homeopathy) was familiar with this mentality, and he said: ". . . *The remarkable and salutary results of the widespread use of Jenner's cowpox vaccine. The smallpox has not since then appeared among us with widespread virulence. Forty or fifty years ago, when a city was stricken, it lost half, often three-quarters of its children."'*

The Council of the Faculty of Homeopathy strongly supports the immunization programme and has stated that immunization should be given in the normal way using conventional tested and approved vaccines.[3] The Society of Homeopathy has no official policy on immunization and says that parents should have full information on efficacy and adverse effects – a view that we support.[14]

These immunizations don't always work. There have been accounts of recent outbreaks of measles and whooping cough where a large proportion of the children who had been immunized still caught the diseases

Unfortunately the reporting of these outbreaks is not always accurate and examination of the facts shows that, in fact, vaccination is highly effective. If 90% of the population is immunized and the vaccine totally ineffective, then you would expect 90% of infected patients to have been vaccinated. This is simply not the case, and the exact degree of protection can be calculated with a standard formula. We do know that a small proportion of people may not make antibodies (protection) with the first injection. For this reason boosters are recommended for certain illnesses, like MMR, because the evidence is that those few who do not make protection first time, will, the second time. For those already protected, the booster will be just that.

How do I know that the vaccines are safe? There's been a lot of publicity that they're not properly tested

All the vaccines currently available have undergone rigorous testing for their effectiveness, safety and the incidence and severity of adverse reactions. No drug – and all vaccines are drugs – can be licensed in this country without proper trials.

Is it safe to take my baby swimming before he is immunized?

Yes, babies may be taken to public swimming pools before receiving their first immunizations. The greatest risk of taking babies swimming is drowning and hypothermia, *not* from a perceived risk of polio infection.

Is it safer to give half a dose of immunization first?

Anything less than the full dose may not give protection. A full dose is as safe as half a dose.

What about rubella vaccine and the fetus?

As a rule, vaccines should not be given to pregnant women unless the risk of getting the infection during the pregnancy outweighs the risk of vaccine damage to the fetus. Under this rule, rubella and other live vaccines are not generally recommended in pregnancy. However, pregnant women have had rubella vaccine inadvertently, and there appears to have been no fetal damage as a result.

What are the chances of my baby being brain damaged from the whooping cough vaccine?

It was not proved that whooping cough vaccine can cause permanent brain damage, but if there is a risk, it is no higher than 1/300 000. There is a much higher risk of damage from catching the disease itself.

Why do I need to have my child immunized if he or she has already had measles or rubella?

Other rashes are often mistaken for measles and rubella and it is therefore better to ensure that each child is fully protected by immunization.

Isn't it immoral to use vaccines derived from aborted fetuses?

This was a much publicized concern in the measles–rubella campaign of 1994. Rubella vaccine was developed by growing viruses on tissue that originated from an aborted fetus, but the abortion was performed for ethical medical reasons and the tissues used for vaccine development were a by-product. Vaccine production does not use any fetal material, and leading religious authorities, particularly those in the Roman Catholic church, said that it was ethical to use rubella vaccines.

10

Future immunization targets

The WHO is aiming to eliminate polio from the world by the year 2000. It also hopes to have stopped neonatal tetanus and congenital rubella by this date. The eradication of measles is a target, but this will require immunization levels over 95%, which may mean two doses for most populations of children.

In many countries, universal hepatitis B vaccination is, or will be, included in the vaccinations given in the first year of life. Some countries (France, for example), offer hepatitis B vaccination in adolescence instead of infancy. This brings vaccination closer to when protection is needed against infection from sexual intercourse and injecting drug misuse. The economic arguments for and against universal hepatitis B vaccination in infancy and adolescence have been well rehearsed.[15] Nevertheless the trend towards combined vaccines and for international vaccine programmes may bring hepatitis B vaccination into the UK schedule.

Meningitis is a more immediate threat to young children. The success of Hib vaccines has strengthened the development of conjugated meningococcal vaccines, for which group A and group C meningococcal vaccines are now in clinical trials in infants in several countries. A group B meningococcal vaccine (needed to prevent 60% of meningococcal infections in Europe and North America) is proving more difficult to produce, but the research is intense. It has been suggested that meningococcal A & C vaccine should be given to university students or other groups of young people. There is no clear strategy that this proposal would be effective, so there is little governmental support.

The re-establishment of the control of diphtheria in Eastern Europe is a high priority. It has brought about the programme of booster doses for teenagers and travellers to Russia and other states in the former Soviet Union.

Pneumococcal vaccines could reduce otitis media and pneumococcal meningitis, and in developing countries could prevent an important cause of chest infections in children. To be effective in children under 2 years of age, the vaccine has to be conjugated, like Hib and the meningococcal vaccines for children. Trials are in progress, with the expectation that there will be a bacterial meningitis vaccine for children.

Varicella (chickenpox) vaccine for children is hotly debated, but the case for giving the vaccine in all children has not yet been clearly established. The vaccine is a live attenuated virus. It is now being used widely in the USA, but it is expensive. The vaccine is not quite as stable as MMR or oral polio, so storage may be a problem. At present, in the UK, varicella vaccine is used for children with leukaemia in whom chickenpox is life-threatening.

Other vaccines under development for children include rotavirus vaccines (to prevent a common cause of infantile gastroenteritis), and a vaccine against respiratory syncytial virus (RSV) which causes bronchiolitis.

There are likely to be vaccines against cancer, either as prevention or as part of the treatment. It could be said that hepatitis B vaccine is already an example of an anti-cancer vaccine, because cancer of the liver is one of the long-term risks of hepatitis B. Vaccines against *Helicobacter pylori* (which causes gastritis and stomach cancer) and other viruses that may cause cervical cancer are other possibilities for the future.

11

Notes on the immune system

The human immune system has evolved to protect people from infections and other substances that could be harmful. It distinguishes between self and non-self and has two important features: its actions are highly specific and the system has memory which provides protection many years after the immunity has been started.

The immune system is complex and this simple account is restricted to vaccines that are given by injection or by mouth. At its very simplest, the immune system produces proteins called antibodies which protect a person against infective organisms and other harmful substances. An antibody works by binding to the harmful substance, broadly termed an 'antigen', and thereby blocks the harmful action of the 'foreign' (non-self) substance.

The antigens that are important in the study of vaccines are the substances produced by micro-organisms, either as toxins or as material that is on, or close to, their outer surfaces. In the earliest vaccines, the antigens were substances naturally produced by micro-organisms. The antigenic substances were inactivated to make them safe for injection. Increasingly in modern times, vaccines have been refined to use purified compounds configured to be antigens. The molecular size of antigens has to be above a certain minimum (in the case of protein antigens, more than 8 amino-acids) to stimulate an immune response.

Antibodies are produced by lymphocytes which are cells that circulate from the lymphatic system into the blood and tissues. The lymphatic system consists of lymph glands that are distributed throughout the body (except in the brain) and lymphatic channels that drain fluids from tissues through lymph glands and into the bloodstream. The lymph glands concentrate lymphocytes and act as filters of antigens.

In early life, the spleen produces blood cells (as does the bone marrow). In older children and adults, the spleen filters antigens and blood cells in the blood stream and concentrates on the destruction of infecting organisms and enhances the production of immunity.

Lymphocytes are divided into two types: B-cells (B because they are derived from bone marrow) and T-cells (derived from the thymus gland). B lymphocytes produce antibody. They can detect antigens in their natural form, but this is not enough on its own to stimulate antibody formation. To do this, B lymphocytes need a stimulus from an important sub-set of T lymphocytes which are called helper cells. In turn, T lymphocytes require another type of cells, called antigen presenting cells, to hold the antigens in a way that T lymphocytes can react to them.

Thus, there is a chain reaction from the introduction of an antigen into the body to the production of antibody. Like other biological processes, this chain is controlled by interactions between cells and the chemicals that they secrete. In general, this is a safety mechanism to prevent unnecessary and harmful reactions. As we learn more about the immune system, so we can use the chain to the advantage and safety of vaccination.

The biochemical substances that promote the formation of antibody after vaccination are called adjuvants. Alum has been used as an adjuvant for diphtheria-tetanus and pertussis vaccine for many years, and it is now known to promote one class of T lymphocyte response – the T helper 2 cells (Th2). As Th2 cells multiply in response to an antigenic challenge, they secrete substances (cytokines) which activate the B lymphocytes and control the activity of other T lymphocytes. Biologically, this may help the immune system to concentrate on specific challenges, whether they be vaccinations or infections. There are adjuvants which promote another class of T lymphocytes – the T helper 1 cells (Th1) which may prove to be better for immunity by vaccination. For this reason, research is being directed to vaccines that favour a Th1 response in preference to a Th2 reaction.

The antibodies produced by lymphocytes are called immunoglobulins (Ig in short) and can be subdivided into various types, with immunoglobulin A (IgA), immunoglobulin G (IgG) and immunoglobulin M (IgM) being of most interest in the defence against infections. IgA antibodies are formed by infections and vaccines that present antigens to the mucosal cells on the inner surfaces of the respiratory and alimentary tracts. IgM antibodies are produced early in the response to antigens that reach the lymphatic system. For medical purposes, the detection of IgM antibody is used as a sign of recent infection or vaccination, typically within the last 3 months. IgG antibody production is more long-term. The circulating antibodies found in blood samples months and years after infection or vaccination are mostly IgG, and IgG antibody production is increased as a defence against a threatened infection.

An individual molecule of IgG lasts for 3 to 9 months in the circulation, if it is not needed to combat infection. This explains why immunity that is transferred across the placenta from mother to baby can protect an infant in the first months of life.

In addition to the highly specific antibody-antigen reactions of the immune system, there are broader defence mechanisms in the immune system. Interferon is produced by lymphocytes (especially T cells) and acts against viruses in a non-specific way, which is why it is used as an anti-viral drug for treating viral hepatitis. During the chain of reaction from antigen presenting cells to antibody production, some of the substances released by lymphocytes and other cells attract macrocytes and polymorphic white blood cells (granulocytes) to the site of inflammation to engulf bacteria and damaged infected cells. This engulfing (phagocytosis) is much more efficient if the micro-organisms have antibody bound to their antigens.

Age has an important effect on the immune system. The immune system is not fully developed by the time a baby is born (biologically this is to ensure that the baby's and mother's immune systems do not harm each other). A newborn baby has sufficient B and T lymphocytes to respond to BCG and hepatitis B vaccines, but not to be immunized by diphtheria-tetanus-pertussis, polio or measles vaccines. By the age of 2 months, the T cells can respond to the protein antigens of DTP, but not the polysaccharide antigens of *Haemophilus influenzae type b*, pneumococci or meningococci unless they are conjugated on to proteins. Maternal IgG antibody may inhibit live viral vaccines given by injection, e.g MMR, but does not stop oral polio vaccine from producing immunity in the intestinal mucosa. By the age of 2 years, the immune system is mature. The thymus gland becomes less active during childhood and ceases to export new lines of T lymphocytes. In older age, immunity depends more and more on immunological memory from childhood and young adulthood, because B lymphocyte production by the bone marrow also falls. For these reasons, a better understanding of the function of the immune system will help the development of vaccines.

References

1 World Health Organization (1985) *Targets for Health for all.* WHO, Copenhagen.
2 Begg N and White J (1987) *A survey of pre-school immunisation programmes in England and Wales.* PHLS Communicable Disease Surveillance Centre, London.
3 DoH (1996) *Immunisation against infectious disease.* HMSO, London.
4 Kulenkampff M, Schwartzman JS and Wilson J (1974) Neurological complications of inoculations. *Arch. Dis. Child.* **49**: 46–9.
5 Office of Health Economics (1984) *Childhood vaccination: current controversies.* OHE London.
6 DHSS (1981) *Whooping cough. Reports from the Committee on Safety of Medicines and the Joint Committee on Vaccination and Immunisation.* HMSO, London.
7 Davies EG, Elliman DAC, Hart CA *et al.* (1996) *Manual of Childhood Infections.* WB Saunders, London.
8 Olin *et al.* (1997) Randomised controlled trial of two-component, three-component and five-component acellular pertussis vaccines compared with whole-cell pertussis vaccine. *Lancet.* **350**: 1569–77.
9 Beck S *et al.* (1991) Egg hypersensitivity and measles/mumps/ rubella vaccine administration. *Paediatrics.* **8(5)**: 913–17.
10 Ingram M (1995) *Managing immunization in general practice.* Radcliffe Medical Press, Oxford.
11 Institute of Medicine (1994) *Adverse events associated with childhood vaccines: evidence bearing on causality.* National Academy Press, Washington.
12 Pollock TM *et al.* (1983) A seven-year study of disorders attributed to vaccination in North West Thames Region. *Lancet.* **i**: 753–7.

13 Bowie C (1990) Lessons from the pertussis vaccine court trial. *Lancet.* **335**: 397–9.

14 Carlyon J (1995) The Society of Homeopathy has no official policy on vaccination. *BMJ.* **310**: 939–40.

15 Health Education Authority (1998) *Health update: immunization.* HEA, London.

Further reading

Brahams D (1988) Pertussis vaccine: Court finds no justification for association with permanent brain damage. *Lancet.* **i**: 837.

Hutchinson T *et al.* (1987) A training procedure for immunisation. *Health Trends.* **19**: 19–24.

Jefferson N *et al.* (1987) Immunisation of children at home without a doctor present. *BMJ.* **294**: 423–4.

Miller CL (1983) Current impact of measles in the United Kingdom. *Rev Infect Dis.* **5**: 427–32.

Miller CL *et al.* (1981) Pertussis immunization and serious acute neurological illness in children. *BMJ.* **282**: 1595–7.

Nicoll A and Rudd P (1989) *British Paediatric Association manual of infections and immunisations in children.* Oxford University Press, Oxford.

Nottingham Community Health NHS Trust (1996) *A practical guide to immunisation in children,* 5th edn. Nottingham Community Health NHS Trust.

Robertson C and Bennett V (1987) Health visitors' views on immunisation. *Health Visitor.* **60**: 221–2.

von Reyn CF *et al.* (1987) Human immunodeficiency virus infection and routine childhood immunisation. *Lancet.* **ii**: 669–72.

Wells N (1987) Immunization – where do we go from here? In (ed. JA Macfarlane) *Progress in child health,* pp. 60–70. Churchill Livingstone, Edinburgh.

Appendix A
Child resuscitation pack

The pack should contain:

- 2 × 1 ml ampoules of adrenaline 1:1000 (1 mg/ml). Instructions on the outside of the box should read: 'For infants and children, adrenaline 1:1000 (1 mg/ml). **Dose to be given slowly, over 10–15 seconds, intramuscularly'.**

Table 4: Recommended adrenaline doses

Age (years)	Dose (ml)
<1	0.05
1	0.1
2	0.2
3–4	0.3
5	0.4
6–10	0.5
11–16	0.7
Adults	1.0 depending on build

- 4 × 1 ml syringes

- 4 × 23 G needles

- specific instruction sheet concerning the treatment of anaphylactic shock in children

- airway/mask suitable for children.

Appendix B
Checklist for home immunization

EACH SESSION

- Vaccine available and in date?
- Resuscitation pack to hand?
- Cool-bag and freezer-pack
- Syringes and 23 G needles
- Sharps box
- Sugar lumps
- Cotton wool
- Spoons
- Plasters
- Forms
- Leaflets

EACH CHILD

- Are there any contraindications or special considerations?

▓ Is the child well?

▓ Were there any reactions following a previous immunization?

▓ Are the records available, has the consent been signed and is the parent happy for the immunization to be given?

▓ Define immunization to be given.

▓ Mention to the parents the possibility of a mild reaction. Advice: tepid sponging or a fan will help to keep the child cool; junior paracetamol; lots to drink.

▓ Record the immunization given on all the appropriate records.

Index